Copyright ©

All rights reserved. No part of reproduced in any form without from the publisher except in the case of brief quotations embodied in critical articles or reviews.

Legal & Disclaimer

The information contained in this book and its contents is not designed to replace or take the place of any form of medical or professional advice; and is not meant to replace the need for independent medical, financial, legal or other professional advice or services, as may be required. The content and information in this book have been provided for educational and entertainment purposes only.

You agree that by continuing to read this book, where appropriate and/or necessary, you shall consult a professional (including but not limited to your doctor, attorney, or financial advisor or such other advisor as needed) before using any of the suggested remedies, techniques, or information in this book.

TABLE OF CONTENTS

INTRODUCTION

SECTION ONE: OVERVIEW

What Is COPD

Types of COPD

What Causes COPD?

Symptoms of COPD

How Is COPD Diagnosed?

COPD Treatment Options

Other Treatment Options

SECTION TWO: MANAGING COPD

What's Life Like With COPD?

Avoiding Shortness Of Breath When Eating

SMOKING AND COPD

Protecting Your Lungs

Protect Your Health

Physical Activity and COPD

COPD and Emotional Health

Recognizing Anxiety and Depression

Getting the Care You Need

SECTION THREE: NUTRITION AND COPD

How Does Food Relate to Breathing?

Nutritional Guidelines

Diet Hints

Benefits of following COPD Nutritional Recommendations

How a COPD Diet Plan Works

What to Eat on a COPD Diet

Cooking Tips

Safety

CONCLUSION

INTRODUCTION

Most people are surprised to learn that the food they eat may affect their breathing. Your body uses food as fuel for all of its activities. The right mix of nutrients in your diet can help you breathe easier. No single food will supply all the nutrients you need—a healthy diet has lots of variety. You and your healthcare team will work out a meal plan just for you. Meeting with a registered dietitian nutritionist (RDN) will help you get on track.

SECTION ONE: OVERVIEW

What Is COPD

The very name of the condition starts to tell you what it's like to have it: Chronic obstructive pulmonary disease (COPD) makes it feel like there's something continually blocking the pathway to your lungs, making it hard to breathe. Although it's considered a disease in itself, COPD is also an umbrella term that incorporates several other breathing-related conditions, including emphysema and chronic bronchitis. To understand COPD, let's begin with a quick lesson about the makeup of your lungs.

- This organ is made up of bronchial tubes, which themselves branch into smaller bronchioles—like a network of roots that split off into smaller roots.
- At the ends of the bronchioles, there are alveoli, miniscule air sacs that cluster together. (Picture the pocketed surface of a raspberry, where each pocket represents an air sac of the alveoli.)
- When you breathe in, the alveoli fill up with air and separate out the oxygen, feeding it into the bloodstream via your capillaries.
- In turn, the capillaries expel carbon dioxide back into the alveoli, and that carbon dioxide

is released when you exhale. It's called gas exchange.

When you're healthy, your body has a whopping 480 million alveoli that function like new balloons—pliable and strong. But when you have COPD, these alveoli can be damaged in different ways.

Types of COPD

Beneath the umbrella of COPD, two major breathing conditions stand out. Let's take a closer look at how your breathing is compromised with the two most common forms of COPD:

Emphysema

When the walls of the alveoli break down, instead of having a bunch of little air sacs, one sac leaches into the next, and you end up with fewer, larger, air sacs. The problem with these larger sacs is that there is less overall surface capacity for oxygen to reach your bloodstream. Plus, the airways throughout the lungs can lose their stretchiness, trapping air inside, which is why emphysema causes shortness of breath.

Chronic Bronchitis

When the bronchial tubes become inflamed or irritated, it can lead to coughing and feeling short of breath. The duration of the bronchitis is important. If you're coughing and producing mucus at least three months at a time for two years in a row, it's considered chronic bronchitis, a type of COPD that is treatable, but not fully reversible.

How serious are these breathing problems? Well, COPD is the fourth leading cause of death in the U.S. More than 16.4 million people have been diagnosed with COPD, although experts believe the true number is much higher (many people don't seek help until the disease has advanced). Let's take a closer look at what's behind this chronic lung condition.

What Causes COPD?

For the majority of Americans, COPD is the result of cigarette smoking. The remaining 25 percent of people can attribute it to air pollution—mainly secondhand smoke and chemical fumes, particularly in places where people cook over open flames and are exposed to cooking oil fumes (so-called biomass fuel exposure). Some asthma sufferers are also diagnosed with COPD, and in this case, treatment can usually reverse the inflammation that causes narrowing in the lung's airways.

Symptoms of COPD

Because COPD symptoms could apply to any number of respiratory illnesses, it can be hard for doctors to isolate the cause. The wheezing and coughing can sound like allergies, and the shortness of breath could just be a result of simply getting older or being out of shape. But a cough that lasts six to eight weeks is considered chronic—a sign that COPD might play a role.

With so many broad symptoms, perhaps it's not surprising that COPD is often misdiagnosed. That's particularly true for women, who account for the majority of people with this condition, even though it's commonly thought of as a "man's disease."

Along with a lingering cough, if any of the symptoms below describes your situation, make a beeline to your doc who may then refer you to a pulmonologist. The most common signs of COPD include:

- Chest tightness
- Chronic coughing—sometimes producing mucus, sometimes not
- Fatigue
- Frequent respiratory infections
- Increased shortness of breath
- Wheezing

If you do have one or more of the symptoms above, it's good to see your doctor sooner than later. Some people may avoid getting help because they're afraid of the stigma surrounding smoking or feel like the disease is their fault. But being a smoker doesn't mean you don't deserve health care, and the longer you wait to have your COPD treated, the more it can advance.

If you are experiencing COPD symptoms, you should not be afraid or ashamed. You're one of millions of Americans in the same boat. There are many treatment options and combinations of drugs. Once you receive the proper diagnosis, you and your doctor can figure out a plan to improve your health and quality of life.

How Is COPD Diagnosed?

Your doctor will start by taking your health history, including finding out about your smoking status (past and present) and exposure to pollutants like secondhand smoke and chemicals. You'll likely also be asked about your symptoms and whether other family members have been diagnosed with COPD.

After that, your doctor will send you for a pulmonary function test to assess lung health. You'll do a spirometry test, which involves blowing air through a mouthpiece and into a machine that determines the amount of air you can exhale and the rate you can expel it. (The machine is also used to determine whether treatments are working, and as a tool to understand how COPD is progressing.)

In the future, the Peak Flow Test, currently used to monitor asthma patients, may also be used to evaluate COPD (studies are underway on its effectiveness for COPD diagnosis). The advantage is that it's simpler to administer and less costly.

Additionally, a chest x-ray or computed tomography (CT) scan can detect emphysema and an arterial blood gas test, which measures how much oxygen is in the blood, and can indicate whether your lungs are doing a good job of oxygenating the body while removing carbon dioxide. Your doctor may want to do further blood work to see if there are other issues going on, such as allergies, that may be contributing to COPD symptoms.

With a diagnosis in hand, your physician may then talk to you about staging your COPD. For many years, pulmonologists used the GOLD Stages, one through four, to describe a person's lung function. The Global Initiative for Chronic Obstructive Lung Disease, which established the system, is moving away from that approach and toward a refined grading system that focuses more on symptoms rather than lung function. The reason: Lung function doesn't always correlate with how a person feels, nor is it great at predicting their outcomes.

The grading system for COPD is letter-based, and looks like this:

- A: less symptoms, low risk
- B: more symptoms, low risk
- C: less symptoms, high risk
- D: more symptoms, high risk

There are several assessment tools available to figure out where you fall on the list. But whatever your grade, don't get hung up on it—it's not like cancer staging in that way. Rather, the grading system helps your doctor think about what therapies should be on the table to help you achieve longer periods without breathlessness, and less exacerbations or flares—times in which the symptoms get bad enough to need outpatient treatment or admission to a hospital.

A COPD diagnosis is a call for action. There are things your medical team can do to help—like prescribing drug therapies and other treatments, and tracking your lung function over time. And there are things you can do, too, to improve your situation.

COPD Treatment Options

There is no cure for COPD, and the approaches to managing this condition will vary depending on your grade and other variables like age and overall health. These are some of the common treatments your doctor might discuss with you:

Quitting Smoking

The single most important thing you can do if you've been diagnosed with COPD is to quit smoking (if you do smoke). Yes, we know, if it were easy you would've done it by now. Nicotine is highly addictive and a tough habit to kick.

If you've tried the cold turkey method without success, don't give up. The FDA has approved several medications in the past few years that are effective in helping people quit smoking. Talk to your doctor about possible quitting aids. Remember, it's crucial to managing your COPD symptoms as well as reducing your risk for other issues like cardiac disease and cancer. The earlier you stop, the more you limit damage to the lungs. And try to avoid secondhand smoke, dust, fumes, or other air pollution.

Changing Your Diet

Your pulmonologist will likely talk with you about maintaining (or adopting) a healthy lifestyle, including cleaning up your diet. COPD can be taxing on the body—the muscles that help you breathe sometimes have to work 10 times harder in someone with the disease in order to make it happen. So you want to fuel them, and the rest of your body, with healthy sources of protein, plus a good helping of fiber and healthy fats. While there is no "COPD diet" per se, the Mediterranean diet is widely accepted for being a balanced way of eating.

However, for some people with COPD, the actual act of eating itself can be difficult and cause shortness of breath. If that happens, a few tips: Chew slowly and take small mouthfuls, pausing to breathe between bites, and have small meals throughout the day. If you find you are losing weight, your doctor may connect you with a nutritionist who can offer guidance.

Exercising More

COPD can trigger a vicious cycle. The less you do, the better you feel, because you don't have to breathe as hard. But living a sedentary lifestyle can have physical repercussions that make COPD worse. Bit by bit, you may feel like your COPD is forcing you to miss out on things like seeing friends and family, in order not to tax your breathing.

Daily physical activity can help combat this, to a certain degree. Exercise builds muscle, and the fitter you are, the less exertion you'll need for everyday tasks. Your doctor will help you put together an exercise program that's tailored to your current level of fitness.

Taking Medication

The goal of medications is to open up the breathing airways and to decrease inflammation. It's not unusual for a person with COPD to have asthma as well, and your pulmonologist is trained in treating both of those conditions at the same time. These are a few meds you may consider:

- Bronchodilators: Delivered via inhalers, these drugs help relax the muscles around your airways, making breathing easier. There are short-acting ones that last a few hours and are used when needed. If your COPD is moderate or severe, your doctor may prescribe a long-acting bronchodilator, which is effective for 12 hours or more and taken daily.
- Glucocorticosteroids: Also delivered via an inhaler, these steroids help reduce inflammation that's affecting the airways.

These medications can be taken together, in different ratios, to fit your needs. You'll work with your doctor to figure out what's right for you, knowing that your dosage and combinations of meds may change over time as your condition changes.

Other Treatment Options

If your COPD is more advanced, your doctor may talk with you about additional interventions to help improve your breathing. Sometimes, it can take a bit of trial and error to figure out the approach that's best for you. If something's not working, don't give up. Eventually, you and your doctor will settle on a system that's most effective.

Pulmonary Rehabilitation

This multidisciplinary approach to COPD treatment includes a customized exercise program that is based on your current abilities and your goals. A pulmonary rehabilitation staff member will teach you how to control the pace of your breathing during exercise to increase stamina and strengthen muscles; over time, you'll be able to exercise for longer.

Pulmonary rehabilitation may also include nurses, physical therapists, respiratory therapists, dieticians, and mental health experts, all of whom will work to put you in charge of your breathing. If you smoke, the program will help in your effort to quit.

Overall, the goal is improving or maintaining lung function for as long as possible. One of the limitations of pulmonary rehabilitation has been around access, including the willingness of insurance companies to cover it, and the effort it takes to attend sessions. Despite its effectiveness, only a small percentage of COPD patients complete a pulmonary rehabilitation program.

Supplemental Oxygen

If your lungs aren't able to supply your bloodstream with enough oxygen, your doctor may outfit you with oxygen therapy.

There are a few different devices that'll do the job, depending on your lifestyle and needs. You breathe it in using an oxygen cannula (a little plastic tube with short prongs that sit just inside your nose) or a face mask. Supplemental oxygen can help you feel better and stay active, which can improve your life overall.

Surgery

For a small number of patients, surgery may be considered. There are a few options.

- Bullectomy: A very small number of patients with emphysema will have air sacs that become extremely large—so called bullae. They take up so much extra space that they prevent healthy air sacs from functioning to their fullest. A bullectomy can remove these giant bullae.

- Lung volume reduction surgery: Other emphysema patients—but again, a small portion—have healthy air sacs in the bottom portion of the lungs, and more damaged air sacs at the top. Lung volume reduction surgery (LVRS) removes the non-functioning portion of lung. But it's a pretty major surgery, so you need to have a relatively high fitness level for this to be eligible for it.
- Endobronchial valve volume reduction: This procedure involves deflating the portion of diseased lung tissue, to allow the healthy

parts to function more effectively. It is a very rare, new, and experimental treatment, and doctors are trying to learn which patients respond well and which don't.

- Lung transplants: These procedures are hardly ever done; patients have to be sick enough to need this extreme intervention, but healthy enough to withstand the surgery (and there's a dearth of organs). While lung transplants won't extend a person's life with COPD, it may increase quality of life.

SECTION TWO: MANAGING COPD

What's Life Like With COPD?

If you've been newly diagnosed with COPD, you may feel overwhelmed and scared. Depression and anxiety are common among patients with COPD, which makes it difficult to commit to the lifestyle changes that can improve your condition. If you're feeling down, tell your pulmonologist or your general practitioner. Together, you can come up with a plan to give your mental health the support it needs. Bonus: Treating mental health is easier than ever with the boom in telemedicine, thanks to the pandemic.

Insurance companies and Medicare are starting to cover more telemedicine, too. There are a lot of people out there ready to support you in whatever ways you need.

In many ways, living with COPD isn't so different than dealing with any other chronic condition: Some days are good, some not-so-great. That's why pulmonary rehabilitation can be so helpful. It's a form of self-management, giving you the knowledge you need to treat your own disease (in concert with what your pulmonologist and other health care providers are doing). That's also why going to your scheduled doctor visits is so important. The "chronic" part of COPD is key here: If you miss out on getting regular medical attention, you could be held back by limitations that are controllable with medication and lifestyle changes.

Avoiding Shortness Of Breath When Eating

One of the symptoms of chronic obstructive pulmonary disease (COPD) is dyspnea, difficulty breathing that often interferes with many activities, including eating. Mealtimes can become frustrating. You may find you feel energy-depleted and malnourished because of this dyspnea, not to mention the sheer physical work it takes to finish eating your food.

If you are finding it difficult to complete your meals because of shortness of breath when eating, try these seven tips. And if this continues to worsen, be sure to mention it to your physician.

Eat for Energy

Because some people with COPD are thin or even malnourished, it's best to choose foods that are high in calories to keep your energy levels soaring, which will positively impact your breathing. Try filling your plate with plant-based fats like coconut, olives, avocado, and nuts and seeds.

Likewise, be sure to include lots of fruits and vegetables in your diet, as they will give you the nutrients you need to fight infection and minimize inflammation.

Choose Easy-to-Chew Foods

Foods that are hard to chew are also difficult to swallow. This puts you at greater risk for choking, aspiration pneumonia, and even death.

Excess chewing can also zap your energy levels during meals, making it impossible for you to finish your meal.

Eating foods that are easy to chew will help you conserve energy so you retain more for breathing. Choosing tender, well-cooked meat, rather than tougher cuts, and well-cooked fruits and vegetables (rather than raw) may help. On the days you are exceptionally fatigued, consider a liquid meal, like a whole-food, protein-rich smoothie, or a liquid meal replacement or nutritional supplement, such as Ensure or Boost.

Opt for Smaller, More Frequent Meals

Eating more frequently means you'll require less food at each sitting, resulting in less labored breathing while you eat. Shifting to smaller meals can also reduce the pressure in your stomach after eating, making it easier to breathe while also reducing the risk of heartburn.

Clear Your Airways Before Dining

Effective airway clearance is an important part of COPD management and can be especially beneficial before meals. When done on a regular basis, airway clearance techniques can help remove sputum (mucus) from the lungs. This can help you breathe more easily and feel better overall.

There are a few different airway breathing techniques you can perform, including:

- Controlled coughing
- Engaging in chest physiotherapy, either manually or with an airway clearance device
- Postural drainage (which is usually coupled with chest physiotherapy)

Go Slow

Eating too fast not only interferes with your digestion and causes you to eat more than you should, but it can drain you of essential energy, making breathing during meals that much more difficult. The next time you sit down to eat, try making your meal last at least 20 minutes.

Take small bites and chew your food slowly. Make a conscious effort to breathe while you are eating. Put your utensils down between bites to ensure that you take your time.

Eat While Sitting Upright

Lying down or slumping while eating can place added pressure on your diaphragm. Proper posture, especially during meal times, will benefit your breathing by keeping excess pressure off your diaphragm, the major muscle of respiration.

Use Pursed-Lip Breathing

Pursed-lip breathing is a breathing technique that is very helpful to use when you become short of breath. It can also help reduce the anxiety associated with dyspnea and allow you to finish a meal.

Perform pursed-lip breathing when you feel short of breath during meals and you may be surprised at what a difference it can make.

To perform pursed-lip breathing, first, relax your shoulders by dropping them down. Then follow these three steps:

1. Take a normal breath through your nose with your mouth closed for two seconds.

2. Pucker your lips like you are about to give someone a kiss or blow out a candle.

3. Very slowly breathe out through your mouth for four seconds.

Save Beverages Until You're Done

When you drink liquids during your meals, you may fill up quickly and feel full or bloated, which can then lead to difficulty breathing. Try waiting until the end of your meal to drink your beverages. But, of course, if you need to sip water while you eat to make food go down easier, do so.

In addition, avoid bubbly drinks, especially sugary sodas, as sugar may cause inflammation and carbonation may worsen your breathing.

SMOKING AND COPD

Smoking is an unhealthy habit for many reasons, not the least of which is that it causes irreversible lung damage that defines chronic obstructive pulmonary disease (COPD). In fact, smoking is the leading cause of this life-threatening pulmonary disease; according to the Centers for Disease Control and Prevention

(CDC), smoking accounts for 80% of all COPD-related deaths.

Once you are diagnosed with COPD, your doctor will strongly suggest that you quit smoking to slow down the progression of your lung disease. In fact, smoking cessation is the most effective strategy for preventing further decline.

Affect on Your Lungs

Among people who smoke, chronic lung disease accounts for 73% of all smoking-related illnesses. In former smokers, chronic lung disease accounts for 50% of all smoking-related conditions. That's because smoking causes a number of different harmful reactions in the lungs. Each of these can contribute to COPD.

When you smoke, your lungs become inflamed. The inflammation damages lung tissue, causing it to thicken. Thickened bronchi (airways) obstruct air as you inhale and exhale, causing the symptoms of COPD. Resulting oxygen deprivation makes you feel short of breath and exhausted, and your risk of lung infections increases.

The harmful chemicals introduced to your lungs when you smoke lead to cellular changes that permanently interfere with your airway expansion and contraction. The resulting lung stiffness further contributes to shortness of breath and exercise intolerance.

Smoking continues to damage the lungs even after COPD develops, worsening the disease and triggering exacerbations (sudden airway narrowing and severe respiratory distress). Exacerbations can be life-threatening and can add to underlying disease severity.

In addition to this, smoking induces an abrupt elevation of chemicals in the blood that are linked with COPD-associated death.

Other Smoking-Related Illnesses

Smoking is a known risk factor for a number of diseases, including lung cancer, heart disease, stroke, breast cancer, stomach cancer, esophageal cancer, and osteoporosis.

Some of these—such as heart disease and lung cancer—cause dyspnea (shortness of breath) and fatigue that amplify the symptoms of COPD.

Each year, 450,000 Americans lose their lives to smoking-related illnesses. This represents one in five deaths, making it the leading preventable cause of death in the U.S.

The Impact of Quitting

Smoking cessation is an important part of managing COPD and of preventing the disease from worsening. People who have COPD and continue to smoke are more likely to need higher medication doses, use urgent rescue inhalers, have more exacerbations, and experience an overall worsening of the disease and a decline in health.

Lung function declines naturally with age, but stopping smoking will slow the decline.

The best time to quit smoking once you are diagnosed with COPD is as soon as possible.

Smoking Cessation: Where to Begin

It's important to recognize that the process of quitting smoking isn't easy while remembering that it is entirely worthwhile. Since quitting can be a challenge, you may be more successful in your efforts if you ask for professional guidance to help you through the process.

There are a variety of cessation strategies you can consider, from using medication to drawing strength from support groups and therapy. Start by talking to your doctor about the best method for you. You might benefit from a carefully designed combination of approaches.

Medication

Your doctor might prescribe nicotine replacement therapy in the form of a patch or a pill to help you avoid nicotine withdrawal symptoms as you work on getting over your smoking habit.

Keep in mind that some prescription medications used in smoking cessation might not be safe for you if you have a systemic disease, such as heart disease or vascular disease.

Therapy

Counseling and behavioral approaches can help you understand your feelings about smoking. You can also learn to shift your mindset and use strategies like meditation to cope with the challenges of smoking cessation.

In fact, mindfulness has been shown to induce changes in the brain that are associated with success in smoking cessation.

Lifestyle Strategies

It might help to make other healthy changes while you are quitting smoking. Exercising keeps you busy and improves your mood, alleviating some of the negative feelings associated with smoking cessation. Keep in mind that if smoking is a social activity for you, exercising with other people can help fill that void. Speak to your doctor before beginning a new exercise routine.

Adding healthy habits like drinking more water and eating nutritious food can help replace the habit of smoking at certain times as well.

Obstacles to Quitting

There are a number of things that get in the way of quitting, including a lack of motivation to quit, enjoying smoking, withdrawal symptoms, and the difficulty of leaving the habit behind.

Acknowledge these challenges and discuss them with your doctor.

Lack of Motivation

There's no question that quitting has to be your choice. You might feel that everyone is telling you to quit smoking, but you might not be so convinced about it yourself.

Smoking cessation is not something that anyone can do for you. You have to do it yourself.

There is an abundant amount of scientific evidence that smoking is harmful. If you are not convinced that it's time to make the change, consider examining how long you plan to continue smoking and make a realistic timeline of the financial and health costs. Your doctor may be able to help with the latter.

Doing this and seeing this information in black and white may help motivate you to see the value in quitting.

Smoking Is a Habit

There may be certain times of the day when you like to smoke, or friends or places that you associate with smoking.

Stopping requires a new mind frame and an acceptance that you can enjoy life even if you don't smoke at specific times, with certain people, or in certain locations.

Giving up a habit often involves replacing it with a new routine—such as walking or knitting or volunteering—with the same friends you used to smoke with or with different friends.

Withdrawal Symptoms

Even if you decide to stop smoking, the withdrawal symptoms—which include irritability, anxiety, jitteriness, trouble concentrating, and changes in appetite—can be unpleasant enough to make you turn back to smoking.

Withdrawal symptoms are temporary, but they can make you feel miserable for days and lag for up to two months. You don't have to put up with these symptoms. Medication and/or anxiety reduction therapy can help minimize or alleviate the effects of nicotine withdrawal.

Smoking Is Comforting for You

The reason that smoking is such a habit-forming addiction is that it induces a sense of enjoyment and relaxation for some people. It can be hard to give that up.

When you are stressed or anxious, you might not have another way to deal with your feelings other than smoking. And you might want to keep getting that enjoyment and pleasure that you get from smoking.

Behavioral therapy or counseling might be helpful as you deal with losing these positive feelings that you get from smoking.

Protecting Your Lungs

The lungs are different from most of the other organs in your body because their delicate tissues are directly connected to the outside environment. Anything you breathe in can affect your lungs. Since the lungs of people who have chronic obstructive pulmonary disease (COPD) are already compromised, reducing your exposure to anything that could make your COPD worse, or cause an exacerbation or flare-up is important.

Avoid Possible Triggers

Smoke: Smoking causes lung cancer, COPD and many other illnesses. To protect your lungs:

- Don't start smoking
- Quit smoking if you smoke
- Avoid secondhand smoke

Industrial Compounds: If you are exposed to dust and fumes at work, ask your health and safety advisor about how you are being protected and talk to your doctor about what can be done to minimize or eliminate the exposure.

Pollution: Help fight pollution. Work with others in your community to help clean up the air you and your family breathe. Get lifesaving updates on your local air quality and learn how you can help fight for healthy air.

Protect Your Health

Taking steps to protect your overall health will also help protect your lungs from viruses and infections that could make you sick.

With COPD, a cold or other respiratory infection can become very serious. There are several things you can do to protect yourself:

- Wash your hands often
- Use hand sanitizer
- Avoids crowds during the cold and flu season

- Ask that extended family members and friends be considerate of your COPD and only visit when they are healthy, which helps you protect yourself from infection.
- Good oral hygiene can stop the germs in your mouth leading to infections. Brush your teeth at least twice a day and see your dentist at least every six months.
- Get vaccinated against flu and pneumonia, and encourage family and those around you to do the same.

Physical Activity and COPD

Regular exercise is part of a healthy lifestyle, even if you have chronic obstructive pulmonary disease (COPD). You might feel like it is not safe, or even possible to exercise, but the right amount and type of exercise has many benefits. Be sure to ask your doctor before you start or make changes to your exercise routine.

Moderate exercise can improve:

- The body's use of oxygen
- Energy levels
- Anxiety, stress and depression
- Sleep
- Self-esteem
- Cardiovascular fitness
- Muscle strength
- Shortness of breath

It might seem odd that exercising when you are short of breath actually improves it—but it works! Exercises help your blood circulate and helps your heart send oxygen to your body. It also strengthens your respiratory muscles. This can make it easier to breath.

Before you start exercising, talk to your doctor about what types and amounts of exercise are right for you.

What Type of Exercises Are Generally Good for People with COPD?

Pulmonary Rehabilitation can be a great way to stay active and learn how to exercise with COPD. This program consists of education and exercise classes that teach you about your lungs and your disease, and how to exercise and be more active with less shortness of breath. The classes take place in a group setting, giving you the chance to meet others with your condition while both giving and receiving support.

Stretching relaxes you and improves your flexibility. It's also a good way to warm up before and cool down after exercising. Practice holding a gentle stretch for 10 to 30 seconds, slowly breathing in and out. Repeat this a few times.

Aerobic exercise is good for your heart and lungs and allows you to use oxygen more efficiently. Walking, biking and swimming are great examples of aerobic exercise. Try and do this type of exercise for about a half an hour a few times a week.

Resistance training makes all your muscles stronger, including the ones that help you breathe. It usually involves weights or resistance bands, but you don't need to go to a gym to do resistance training. Ask your doctor or respiratory therapist to show you some exercises you can do at home. To get stronger, do these exercises three to four times a week.

It is generally safe for people with COPD to exercise but you should not exercise if:

- You have a fever or infection

- Feel nauseated
- Have chest pain
- Are out of oxygen

Contact your doctor right away if you are experiencing any of these symptoms.

Should I Use My Oxygen When I Exercise?

If you use supplemental oxygen, you should exercise with it. Your doctor may adjust your flow rate for physical activity, which will be different than your flow rate when you are resting. Work with your doctor to adjust your oxygen for physical activity.

Here are some other tips for breathing during exercise:

- Remember to inhale (breathe in) before starting the exercise and exhale (breathe out) through the most difficult part of the exercise.
- Take slow breaths and pace yourself.
- Purse your lips while breathing out.

Ways to Stay Active

- Try to get up and out each day, even just to walk to another room, take a shower or get the mail. Every little bit helps.
- Light stretching is a great way to stay mobile and avoid over exertion.
- Participate in activities you enjoyed before you were diagnosed. You may need to modify them, but they can still be enjoyed.

- Set achievable goals for yourself such as taking a short walk every day.
- Check out exercise programs on your television, online or cellphone apps.
- Participate in a pulmonary rehabilitation program.

COPD and Emotional Health

For people living with COPD, the physical challenges of managing the disease can sometimes affect their mood and emotional health. Most COPD patients experience feelings of sadness, fear and worry at times. This is common and normal when coping with a serious illness. But if those feelings don't go away after a few weeks, or they start to affect your ability to keep up with normal activities and enjoy life, then you may be experiencing symptoms of anxiety or depression.

Recognizing Anxiety and Depression

Anxiety and depression are both more common in people living with COPD than they are in the general population, but unfortunately, they often go unrecognized and untreated by patients, caregivers and healthcare providers. Taking care of your emotional health does more than just improve your mood. Research shows that managing anxiety and depression can increase your ability to stick with your prescribed COPD treatment, improve your physical health and reduce medical costs.

Clinical anxiety is defined as constant worrying and anticipating the worst in a way that makes it hard to function. For people living with COPD, shortness of breath can cause anxiety and even panic attacks. Anxiety makes you breathe faster, which increases your shortness of breath. Experiencing worry about avoiding shortness of breath can make you less active, which in turn can worsen your fitness. When we are active, we strengthen our lungs, so becoming less active can make shortness of breath worse. Staying active can also have positive effects on our mental health, which can help keep anxiety and depression at bay.

Clinical depression is a feeling of deep sadness or emptiness that lasts longer than a couple of weeks. It affects your ability to enjoy your work, recreation, family and friends. Depression is a serious illness that affects more than just your mood.

Things You Can Do

Although anxiety and depression are common in people with COPD, they do not have to be inevitable and should never be ignored. There are positive steps you can take to help yourself feel better.

1. Talk to your healthcare team about your mood. Ask them to work with you to understand the cause of your feelings, and to identify coping strategies that will work for you. They may recommend you speak with a mental health professional such as a counselor, psychologist or psychiatrist.

There are medications available to help with anxiety and depression, but they have not always been found to be effective for people with COPD. Counseling, or talk therapy, can successfully help people living with COPD change patterns of negative thinking and behaviors, improve quality of life and reduce anxiety and depression.

2. Take care of yourself. Even though you may not feel like it, staying active is well worth the effort for both your body and your mind. Try to see friends, get outside and keep doing the things that you enjoy as best you can. Exercise can help clear your mind and lighten your mood.

Manage your stress and reduce the feeling of shortness of breath by practicing relaxation techniques and breathing exercises. Writing in a journal or working on a coloring book can help you process your feelings and quiet your mind.

Ask for help when you are feeling isolated or overwhelmed. Most people in your life want to help, but they don't know how. Don't be afraid to ask your friends, family, neighbors and care team to help you through hard times.

3. Connect with others who understand what it's like to live with COPD. Look for a Better Breathers Club or other COPD support group in your area. Going to meetings has the added benefit of getting you out of the house. You can also join an online support community like the Living with COPD Community on Inspire, to get free expert

information and referral to resources from a nurse or respiratory therapist.

If You Are a Caregiver

Sometimes the best thing you can do as a caregiver is to listen. It might be tempting to try to problem solve, but sometimes just lending an ear is the best medicine. However, don't be afraid to suggest your loved one talk to a professional and call the doctor immediately if you believe they are a danger to themselves.

The stress of caring for a loved one with COPD can take a toll on your own mental and emotional health. As a caregiver, it is normal to struggle at times with feelings of anger, frustration and guilt. To avoid being overwhelmed, it is important to take the time to care for your own health and well-being.

Planning for the Future with COPD

Being diagnosed with a chronic disease like chronic obstructive pulmonary disease (COPD) can make you and your caregivers think about uncomfortable topics you may not have explored before, including long-term, palliative and even hospice care. Thinking through these potential situations now and discussing your wishes with your loved ones helps ensure that you will get the care you want in the future.

Getting the Care You Need

Palliative, or supportive care, is aimed at making you more comfortable and improving your quality of life. Prescription medications may be offered to relieve your physical and emotional symptoms amd counseling is available to support your emotional and/or spiritual well-being. Palliative care can also help by addressing practical concerns such as care coordination and life-planning.

Sometimes people confuse palliative care with hospice care. Hospice care is given at the end-of-life while palliative care is appropriate at any stage of your disease. Talk to your doctor about any physical or emotional concerns you may have. Then you can work together to get the supportive care you need while planning for the care you want in the future.

Points for Discussion

There may come a time when you cannot communicate your wishes. For this reason, it is important to discuss them ahead of time with your family or friends, and fill out the appropriate paperwork (advance directives) as early as possible. The sooner you discuss what you want, the less stressful it will be for you and your support system if the time comes when they may have to make potentially difficult decisions. Use the topics below as guidelines for talking to your caregivers and doctors about end-of-life care. There are many other topics that will be addressed in advance directive. The doctor can help you get an advance directive form. Your healthcare team can help you navigate this difficult yet important decision making.

Getting Paperwork in Order

- Create an advance directive. An advance directive consists of two documents: Healthcare Power of Attorney, and Living Will.
    - A healthcare power of attorney designates someone you know and trust

to make healthcare decisions for you if you are unable to do so yourself.
- A living will outlines your end-of-life medical care choices. Your healthcare power of attorney can use this document to guide their decisions and put a voice to your wishes, rather than having to make decisions themselves. This can make it easier to honor your wishes.

• Work with an estate-planning attorney, or your local legal aid office, to draft a durable financial power of attorney to appoint someone you trust to make decisions about your finances; this person will also have access to your assets and accounts.

- Put your financial records in order and store them all in one place (includes account numbers, investments, credit cards, loads, deeds and more)
- Draft your will. This is a document that can be drafted with or without an attorney, and typically consists of where your belongings will go at the end of your life.

Please note: Some states require these documents be notarized, while others do not. Be sure to check the requirements of your state.

There are many other topics that will be addressed in end-of-life planning, and the documents can differ by state. Keep in mind, your doctor's office can provide you with an advance directive, and they are also available online through your state's website. Do not hesitate to rely on your healthcare team, as well as legal counsel (legal aid or private) to help you navigate these difficult, yet important decisions.

SECTION THREE: NUTRITION AND COPD

How Does Food Relate to Breathing?

The process of changing food to fuel in the body is called metabolism. Oxygen and food are the raw materials of the process, and energy and carbon dioxide are the finished products. Carbon dioxide is a waste product that we exhale.

The right mix of nutrients in your diet can help you breathe easier.

Metabolism of carbohydrates produces the most carbon dioxide for the amount of oxygen used; metabolism of fat produces the least. For some people with COPD, eating a diet with fewer carbohydrates and more fat helps them breathe easier.

The right mix of nutrients in your diet can help you breathe easier.

Nutritional Guidelines

Choose complex carbohydrates, such as whole-grain bread and pasta, fresh fruits and vegetables.

- To lose weight: Opt for fresh fruits and veggies over bread and pasta for the majority of your complex carbohydrates.
- To gain weight: Eat a variety of whole-grain carbohydrates and fresh fruits and vegetables.

Limit simple carbohydrates, including table sugar, candy, cake and regular soft drinks.

Eat 20 to 30 grams of fiber each day, from items such as bread, pasta, nuts, seeds, fruits and vegetables. Eat a good source of protein at least twice a day to help maintain strong respiratory muscles. Good choices include milk, eggs, cheese, meat, fish, poultry, nuts and dried beans or peas.

• To lose weight: Choose low-fat sources of protein such as lean meats and low-fat dairy products.

• To gain weight: Choose protein with a higher fat content, such as whole milk, whole milk cheese and yogurt.

Choose mono- and poly-unsaturated fats, which do not contain cholesterol. These are fats that are often liquid at room temperature and come from plant sources, such as canola, safflower and corn oils.

- To lose weight: Limit your intake of these fats.
- To gain weight: Add these types of fats to your meals.

Limit foods that contain trans fats and saturated fat. For example, butter, lard, fat and skin from meat, hydrogenated vegetable oils, shortening, fried foods, cookies, crackers and pastries.

Note: These are general nutritional guidelines for people living with COPD. Each person's needs are different, so talk to your doctor or RDN before you make changes to your diet.

Check Your Weight

Get in the habit of weighing yourself regularly. The scale will alert you to weight loss or gain. You should see your doctor or dietitian if you continue to lose weight or if you gain weight while following the recommended diet. There are health complications that can result from being underweight or overweight. A well-nourished body is better able to handle infections. When people with COPD get an infection, it can become serious quickly and result in hospitalization. Good nutrition can help prevent that from happening. If illness does occur, a well-nourished body can respond better to treatment.

Vitamins and minerals

Many people find taking a general-purpose multivitamin helpful. Often, people with COPD take steroids. Long-term use of steroids may increase your need for calcium. Consider taking calcium supplements. Look for one that includes vitamin D. Calcium carbonate or calcium citrate are good sources of calcium. Before adding any vitamins to your daily routine, be sure to discuss with your doctor.

Sodium

Too much sodium may cause edema (swelling) that may increase blood pressure. If edema or high blood pressure are health problems for you, talk with your doctor about how much sodium you should be eating each day. Ask your RDN about the use of spices and herbs in seasoning your food and other ways you can decrease your sodium intake.

Fluids

Drinking plenty of water is important not only to keep you hydrated, but also to help keep mucus thin for easier removal. Talk with your doctor about your water intake. A good goal for many people is 6 to 8 glasses (8 fluid ounces each) daily. Don't try to drink this much fluid at once; spread it out over the entire day. Some people find it helpful to fill a water pitcher every morning with all the water they are supposed to drink in one day. They then refill their glass from that pitcher and keep track of their progress during the course of the day. Remember, any healthy caffeine-free fluid counts toward your fluid goal, and most foods contribute a substantial amount of fluid, as well.

Using medical nutritional products

You may find it difficult to meet your nutritional needs with regular foods, especially if you need a lot of calories every day. Also, if your RDN has suggested that you get more of your calories from fat—the polyunsaturated, monounsaturated, and low-cholesterol variety—you may not be able to meet this goal easily with ordinary foods. Your RDN or doctor may suggest you drink a liquid called a medical nutritional product (supplement). Some of these products can be used as a complete diet by people who can't eat ordinary foods, or they can be added to regular meals by people who can't eat enough food.

Diet Hints

- Rest just before eating.
- Eat more food early in the morning if you're usually too tired to eat later in the day.
- Avoid foods that cause gas or bloating. They tend to make breathing more difficult.
- Eat 4 to 6 small meals a day. This enables your diaphragm to move freely and lets your lungs fill with air and empty out more easily
- If drinking liquids with meals makes you feel too full to eat, limit liquids with meals; drink an hour after meals.

- Consider adding a nutritional supplement at night time to avoid feeling full during the day

Benefits of following COPD Nutritional Recommendations

COPD is a lung disease that causes a number of symptoms, including dyspnea (shortness of breath) and fatigue due to airway inflammation and narrowing.

There are a variety of benefits when it comes to following nutritional recommendations in COPD. Weight control, keeping your immune system healthy, helping your lungs heal from damage, maintaining your energy, and avoiding inflammation are among the ways your diet can enhance your health when you have this disease.

These effects won't reverse the condition, but they can help keep it from getting worse.

Weight Control

Weight is complicated when it comes to COPD. Obesity is considered a COPD risk factor. And being overweight places a high demand on your heart and lungs, making you short of breath and worsening your COPD symptoms.

But malnutrition and being underweight can pose a major problem in COPD too.2 Chronic disease puts increased demands on your body, robbing your body of nutrients. And, a lack of nutrients makes it even harder for you to heal from the recurrent lung damage inherent with COPD.

This means that weight control is something you need to be serious about. Regularly weighing yourself can help you get back on track quickly if you veer away from your ideal weight range. Strategic diet choices, of course, can help you stay on track.

Strengthening Your Immune System

Any infection, especially a respiratory one, can make it difficult to breathe and can lead to a COPD exacerbation.

When you have COPD, a pulmonary infection has a more severe impact on your already impaired lungs. And COPD itself results in a diminished ability to avoid infections through protective mechanisms like coughing.

Getting adequate nutrients like protein, vitamin C, and vitamin D through diet can help your immune system fight off infections.

Healing From Damage

Recurrent lung damage is the core problem in COPD. When your body is injured, it needs to heal. Nutrients like vitamin E and vitamin K help your body repair itself.

Maintaining Energy

COPD leads to low energy. You need to consume carbohydrates to fuel yourself.

Iodine, an essential mineral, helps your body make thyroid hormone to regulate your energy metabolism. Your body also needs adequate vitamin B12 and iron to keep your oxygen-carrying red blood cells healthy.

Avoiding Inflammation

Inflammation plays a major role in COPD. Experts recommend a diet rich in antioxidants such as plant-based foods and omega-3 fatty acid-rich seafood to help combat excessive inflammation.

Research also suggests that artificial preservatives may induce an inflammatory response that promotes diseases such as COPD, so they should be avoided.

How a COPD Diet Plan Works

A COPD diet plan is fairly flexible and can include many foods that you like to eat. General guidelines include:

- Avoiding allergy and asthma triggers
- Eliminating (or at least minimizing) processed foods
- Including fruits, vegetables, beans, nuts, dairy, lean meats, and seafood

You can follow a vegetarian or vegan diet if you want to, but you will need to make sure that you get enough fat and protein by eating things like avocados and healthy oils.

Duration

A COPD diet is meant to be followed for a lifetime. This is a chronic, incurable disease, and following these diet guidelines consistently can help you manage symptoms along the way.

What to Eat on a COPD Diet

There are plenty of options you can include in your diet when you have COPD. If you're having a hard time coming up a nutrition plan that is to your liking, a dietitian can help.

Fruit and Vegetables

Fresh or cooked fruits and vegetables are resources for essential vitamins and minerals. They also contain natural antioxidants that help promote healing and counteract inflammation. Consider the wide array of options, including potatoes, beets, spinach, carrots, broccoli, asparagus, bananas, peaches, blueberries, and grapes.

Energy-Rich Carbohydrates

You need a daily supply of energy, most of which comes from carbohydrate calories. Complex carbohydrates like whole grains can give you lasting energy. Simple carbohydrates like candy can give you a burst of energy, but then the excess calories are quickly stored as fat (leading to weight gain).

Consuming too much carbohydrate calories can lead to obesity and may increase your risk of diabetes. On the other hand, not consuming enough can leave you low in energy and underweight.

Make sure you get some professional guidance regarding your optimal calorie intake, which is calculated based on your age and height. Your COPD will also be considered, as it may mean that your body has a higher energy requirement.

According to the American Lung Association, your breathing muscles may need 10 times as many calories if you have COPD than breathing muscles of a person without the disease.

Proteins and Fats

Proteins are vital to your healing process, and they also help your body make immune cells. Foods like seafood, beef, poultry, pork, dairy, eggs, and beans contain protein.

Fats help you digest your food and make vitamins. Foods like meat, dairy, eggs, nuts, and oils contain fat.

Fiber

It's important to include enough fiber in your diet. While you might already know that fiber keeps your bowel movements regular and helps protect against colon cancer, a diet high in fiber is also associated with better lung function and reduced respiratory symptoms in people with COPD.

High-fiber foods include vegetables, legumes (beans and lentils), bran, whole grains, rice, cereals, whole-wheat pasta, and fresh fruit. These foods are also anti-inflammatory.[1]

Your fiber consumption should be between approximately 21 and 38 grams of fiber each day, depending on your age and gender.[7]

Beverages

Unless your doctor tells you otherwise, you should drink six to eight eight-ounce glasses of water daily. This helps to keep your mucus thin, making it easier to cough up.

It's easy to forget to drink, especially if you haven't been in the habit of hydrating. You might consider filling a large water bottle with your daily fluid requirements every morning and sipping on it throughout the day.

If plain water isn't palatable to you, and try warm or chilled herbal or green tea.

Alcohol can make you tired, especially if you are already chronically low in energy. And caffeine can raise your blood pressure or cause heart palpitations, making you feel light-headed, dizzy, or shorter of breath than usual. As some people with COPD may feel worse after consuming alcoholic or caffeinated beverages, it may be best to avoid or limit these.

Recommended Timing

Small, frequent calorie-dense meals can help you meet your caloric needs more efficiently if you are having a hard time keeping weight on. Small meals can also help you feel less full or bloated, making it more comfortable to breathe deeply.

Avoiding Shortness of Breath While Eating

Cooking Tips

You might enjoy keeping track of calories, reading nutrition labels, and coming up with new recipes. But not everyone wants to focus so much on every dietary detail or spend time working on creating a meal plan.

If you prefer to follow specific instructions for a personalized menu, talk to your doctor about getting a consultation with a nutritionist or a dietitian. You can get recipes or guidelines from a professional and ask questions about how to modify dishes to your preferences and for your disease.

Cooking guidelines to keep in mind include:

- Avoid deep-frying your food: This process creates trans fats, which can lead to additional cellular damage in your lungs beyond the damage that's already there due to COPD.

- Use salt in moderation: This is especially important if you have high blood pressure or edema (swelling of the feet or legs). Edema is a late-stage complication of COPD.
- Use fresh herbs to add natural flavor, which can reduce your reliance on salt.
- Use natural sweeteners like honey, ginger, or cinnamon instead of sugar. Excess sugar can increase the risk of edema.

Modifications

One of the most important dietary guidelines to keep in mind when you have COPD is avoiding foods that may trigger an allergic reaction or an asthma attack.

Allergies and asthma attacks can cause severe, sudden shortness of breath. Anything that triggers a bout of breathing problems can be life-threatening for you when you already have COPD.

Common food triggers include dairy products, eggs, nuts, or soybeans.

You don't need to avoid an allergen (a substance that causes an allergic reaction) if it doesn't cause you to have symptoms, but try to be observant about patterns and trends that exacerbate your symptoms.

If you notice that certain foods affect your breathing, it's important to be vigilant about avoiding them.

Considerations

The basics of a COPD diet are healthy guidelines for everyone. Because of your COPD, however, there are some additional things you should keep in mind when working to follow your eating plan.

Safety

Your tendency to cough when you have COPD could place you at risk of choking when you eat or drink. Be sure to give yourself ample time to consume your food and liquids carefully. Avoid talking while you are eating and drinking so you can reduce your risk of choking.

Shortness of breath can be a problem when eating too. Pace yourself and stick to foods that are not difficult for you to chew and swallow.

If you are on continuous oxygen therapy, make sure you use it while you eat. Since your body requires energy to eat and digest food, you will need to keep breathing in your supplemental oxygen to help you get through your meals.

CONCLUSION

Eating should be a pleasurable activity, and nutrition is an essential component of living well with COPD. If you are finding it difficult to eat because of shortness of breath from your lung condition, speak with your doctor in addition to trying these strategies. You may need to be tested for supplemental oxygen use and you may benefit from seeing a dietitian or nutritionist.

Although a healthy diet cannot cure COPD, it can help you feel better and it can help prevent your disease from getting worse. A COPD diet is flexible and does not cause any adverse side effects or interfere with any of your medications.

Printed in Great Britain
by Amazon